The Power of Meditation
Clear Your Head with Meditation
and Manage Stress while
Improving Concentration and
Clarity

Table of Contents

What is Meditation and how does it Work?

It is a common misconception that meditation is an act of worship or prayer. In reality, 'meditation' as a concept simply means 'awareness'. Any activity you engage in that involves you being actively aware has a meditative quality. For example, slowing your breath is meditation, or listening to the birds singing is meditation. In order for such activities to be 'effective' meditation, they must be free from any other mental distractions.

Do not think of meditation as a technique to learn; meditation is a way of life. It can be described as a principle of ceasing the processes of thought. Once achieved, this state of consciousness liberates a person from the chaos of scattered thoughts they are usually subjected to. Through heightened awareness, an individual is able to reduce all the myriad mental activities down to one focused mentality.

In an experiment for scientific research, a Tibetan Lama allowed himself to have his brain function monitored during deep meditation. The scientist involved was impressed by what he saw, and commented that the Lama was able to achieve a deep mental relaxation, thus validating the effectiveness of his meditation. The Lama corrected the scientist, saying that it was his own mind that validated the effectiveness of the machine that monitored it.

It is not unnatural to think of meditation as a spiritual practice, in which one sits with eyes closed, attempting to achieve enlightenment or perhaps have an experience of the Divine. Some people claim that gardening is their form of meditation, or other mind-focusing activities like exercise, painting or music. These suggestions can lead to confusion or misunderstanding of the very specific, true meaning of meditation.

The word is derived from a pair of Latin words: '*meditari*', meaning '*to think*' or '*to exercise the mind*'; and '*mederi*', meaning '*to heal*'. The Sanskrit origin of the word – '*medha*' - roughly translates as 'wisdom'.

It had been thought for much of the twentieth century – particularly in Western culture – that meditation is something outdated and irrelevant to modern society, but it has had a recent surge in people recognising its value, and that the previous assumption was simply not true. There have been a number of published scientific and medical studies that demonstrate many of its benefits, but there are still aspects of it that remain mysterious in their wondrous effects on people.

Classically, in line with the Buddhist and Yogic traditions, it is believed that in order to attain a true state of meditation one must go through several stages. After establishing the necessary elements of personal and social principles, body position, breath control and relaxation, one must tackle the more complex stages of concentration, contemplation and, finally, absorption. But there is no doctrine that says the order in which one must perfect each of these stages; true meditation is achieved when a person can apply a portion of every element simultaneously.

To the layman, making reference to meditation will often mean finding a way to achieve just one of those elements. Some schools or groups only teach concentration techniques, or relaxation exercises, while others try to push students on to the more advanced techniques before they achieve an understanding of the basics. Many try to sever the association of meditation with yoga for fear that it will be branded 'Eastern'. The reality is that whether you consider it 'Eastern' or not, yoga and its principles are universally relevant to mankind, and without adhering to yoga principles one cannot achieve true meditation.

This doesn't necessarily have to mean learning to contort your body into shapes that require enormous strength and flexibility. It simply means that through regular practice of certain techniques and adherence to the right principles and disciplines, the energy of body and mind can be liberated, expanding the quality of consciousness exponentially! This claim is not a subjective one; the discipline and dedication required is extremely challenging, but the physiological and psychological benefits are becoming increasingly demonstrable by the scientific community.

The health benefits you can expect to enjoy through successful meditation include stress reduction, improved memory, superior concentration and even an expanded creativity and sense of compassion for others. It may seem farfetched that merely learning to control the chaos of thought processes in the mind can yield such a range of benefits. The growing body of scientific evidence that demonstrates the facts is becoming increasingly available for your perusal. Remember to research findings that relate to the holistic, traditional methods of meditation which we call 'mindfulness meditation' or 'focused attention'.

The concept of 'mindfulness' means that practitioners strive to focus their entire mind on a single thought. It is important that an overarching goal must be stoutly applied to the present moment. The typical method taught to students of this meditation is to focus entirely on the breath; one must merely be attentive to each exhalation and inhalation without the interruption of any stray thoughts. If an external thought threatens to arise, the accomplished practitioner will be able to quickly recognise and eliminate it. This doesn't have to be done by focusing on the breath; some focus on other singular thoughts, such as reciting a mantra.

This instruction to be completely singular in your thoughts, inattentive to anything but the individual focus you have chosen, is incredibly difficult to follow, particularly in a modern environment that taxes our attention spans so diversely. Minds are very naturally led to wander from thought to thought; it is actually difficult to go even a few seconds without the arrival of a new thought. Focused attention, over a prolonged period of time, is extremely challenging and cannot be spontaneously achieved. One must practice.

Clearly, the notions that meditation is just a process of chilling out, or even cleansing the mind of all thought, are not accurate. Meditation is a process that requires hard, active work throughout, and cannot be achieved without a great deal of practice. But, as you become more accomplished and experienced in your meditation techniques, you will find that it becomes easier to remain focused. Progress is measured simply by how long a single thought can be focused upon without straying; but you can't allow yourself to be thinking about beating your personal record as you're meditating!

The principle is astoundingly simplistic, but remarkably difficult to achieve. And it yields an equally astonishing number of benefits for such a seemingly simple action. As its popularity continues to soar, scientists become more eager to explore the cognitive effects of meditation, and continue studies with Buddhist monks and Yogis around the world.

Keep in mind that although our considerations in this chapter primarily describe focused attention, there are benefits to other meditative practices, such as open attention, as well.

Changes to the Brain

Meditation has been part of Buddhism for literally millennia. Monks are raised in the tradition of its positive effects, particularly its power to bolster one's inner strength and gain the insight required for extensive spiritual practice. In short, meditation is to Buddhist monks what prayer is to Christians. The key difference, however, is that while Christians are attempting to connect with the presence of Divinity, Buddhists seek a profound connection with their inner self, in order to harness the full power of the mind under total control.

With relatively recent advances in technology, neuroscientists have been able to look directly into the brains of practitioners to get a physical look at how meditation affects brain activity. For example, by using MRI scanning apparatus, neuroscientists have been able to observe that meditation strengthens the brain by reinforcing connections between brain cells. A study in 2012 demonstrated that advanced meditation practitioners exhibit enhanced levels of gyrification (the 'folding' of the cerebral cortex which occurs as the result of physical growth) which potentially enables the brain to act faster than it otherwise would. Scientists theorize that gyrification enhances the brain's capacity for decision making, memory forming and concentration.

The physical changes that occur in the brain as a result of meditation can also have other beneficial implications. Increased cortical thickness, for example, can result in decreased sensitivity to pain and greater resistance to damage. Furthermore, it is thought that long-term meditation can increase the density of gray matter in the brain stem, which can lead to improved cognitive, emotional and immune responses as it positively impacts cardiorespiratory control (our breathing and heart rate). Meditation has also demonstrated neuroprotective capabilities; it can decrease age-related decline in gray matter and cognitive function.

There have been observed differences between meditators and healthy non-meditators in the expression of certain brain metabolites that are linked to conditions such as anxiety and depression. This is galvanized further by the positive effects on general brain activity associated with meditation: the practice of focused attention can lead to decreased default mode network activity and connectivity – those pesky brain activities that cause our concentration to lapse and can lead to disorders such as ADHD and anxiety – and even strengthen the brain's resistance to a build-up of the beta amyloid plaques associated with Alzheimer's disease.

Finally, meditation has been demonstrated to significantly impact electrical brain activity, increasing Theta and Alpha EEG motion, resulting in a highly-developed capacity for wakeful and relaxed attention in day-to-day activities.

Chapter 1 - The Breath and Body Connection

The average person will almost instinctively hold their breath during an act of intense concentration. For example, while attempting to keep a steady hand to win a game, or while balancing on a ledge over a large precipice, a person will naturally hold their breath. In other words, when we are engaging in some important, intense activity that requires our full attention, we automatically dismiss breathing as something non-essential and thus hold our breath. It is very difficult to concentrate on controlling our breathing whilst our full attention is demanded by something else, so although we don't consciously choose to hold our breath, that is exactly what happens.

This demonstrates the relationship between breath and thought. When our entire being is being called upon to focus on something, other functions are temporarily suspended. This is not just limited to the breath; the senses become suspended during those moments as well, meaning other sounds, smells or movements surrounding us can be unnoticed due to the fact that all our attention is focused elsewhere. Essentially, the concentration of the mind, the suspension of breath and the withdrawal of senses all occur simultaneously.

While this state is usually involuntary, and only occurs under exceptional circumstances, it is actually a similar disposition that we aim for during focused attention meditation. There is a story in yoga stating that the complex energies of body and spirit are so intrinsically connected to that of the mind that the stoppage of breath is what brings the mind to its 'normal' condition. The mind is being pulled in opposite directions by its tendencies to pleasure and pain; intense joviality and intense despair are the two extremes between which the mind typically dwells. Whatever state the mind is in, the energies of body and spirit are carried alongside it.

Imagine a bird whose foot is tied with a length of string to a peg. As the bird attempts to escape, it severs the string's connection to the peg and is thus made to carry the string with it wherever it travels. This connection is the same as that of the mind and the breath. The activity of the mind is reflected by the motion of the breath; and one cannot function effectively without the other. Another analogy to describe this relationship is that of a functioning mechanical watch. The mechanism moves the hands, but if the movement of those hands is obstructed then the mechanism itself is unable to function. If either the clockwork mechanism or the movement of the hands is obstructed, then neither is able to function. Such is the relationship between the mind and the breath.

The Retention of Breath

Remember that in meditation, the cessation of unwanted brain function is actually the objective. It is said, in yoga, that a deep exhalation followed by retention of this breathless state can bring about balance in the thinking process. Any external agitation to the mind is expelled from it, at least temporarily, if we attempt to hold our breath with empty lungs for as long as possible. Repeating this process for a period of a few minutes is said to be sufficient for the mind to grow accustomed to the cessation of function, and therefore cease its agitation from external burdens. The same results can be achieved by holding the breath after a deep inhalation, but it is likely to take longer that way.

The techniques of inhaling or exhaling deeply, then retaining a non-breathing state, are two of the four types of *kumbhaka* (breath retention) exercises. The third type is that of alternative breathing, meaning the practitioner breathes in deeply through the left nostril, then retains the breath briefly before exhaling through the right. Retaining the exhaled state, then returning to an inhalation through the left nostril, the practitioner has completed one round of this breathing meditation exercise. The nature of this third kumbakha technique means that it incorporates something of the first two, but is easier to practice as it is less demanding on the respiratory system than the intense first two exercises.

The fourth technique is the most important of the exercises, and is therefore seen to be of most consequence to yoga practice. It is generally achieved through practice of the other three techniques, and is the culmination of them; extended practice of the previously described techniques can give you total control over your breath. Finally you reach a state where you can automatically suspend your breath, without any inhalation or exhalation to prepare, for as long as is necessary. This will mean that if you are suddenly caught off guard by something, you are able to instantly and instinctively cease the breath in order to avoid the onset of chaos in the mind and ensure total concentration on the matter at hand. Only through this retention of breath can you achieve the highest levels of concentration you require. At a highly advanced state, you may have witnessed people who are able to set world records for holding the breath underwater. Through such complete control over the breath, people can slow the heart rate and remain submerged without breathing apparatus for as much as 18 minutes at a time!

When practicing meditation techniques to achieve this fourth state, you will be encouraged to emphasise concentration of the mind over consciously trying to cease breath, as the cessation of breath will happen by itself if the mind is sufficiently focused. As previously stated, if our concentration is intense and all-encompassing, other functions will cease and the surrounding elements will cease to interfere. The link between mind and breath is so profoundly entwined that it is difficult to say where one ends and the other begins. When both are called upon entirely, such as in a period of extreme concentration on a single thing, neither will function; in other words, breathing will cease and the chaotic hyperactivity of the mind will do the same.

It is here that there is some disagreement about the mind-body relationship. Behaviourists and materialists contend that the mind is a slave to the reflexes of bodily functions, and merely a by-product of bodily energy. Idealists, however, contend that the body is under the control and regulation of the mind. This philosophical dispute has endured through the centuries, with neither side truly reaching any definitive conclusions. In yoga, the belief is that neither the materialists nor the idealists are entirely correct about whether it is mind or body that governs everything. Instead, it is more the case that both elements run parallel to one another towards a common destination, with neither being fully responsible for its counterpart as in the case of two legs walking. The yoga practitioner sees purpose in transcending those two walking legs to find what it is that maintains the balance that allows them to function in perfect harmony.

In other words, perhaps there is some transcendent force acting upon body and mind, and the quest to find whether body or mind is the dominant factor is a fool's errand. This higher state acts with purpose and design, and is the state which yoga practitioners wish to gain access to, as it would transcend the necessity to choose a side in philosophical debate in favour of an insight that encompasses all sides at the same time. The limitation of philosophy is that it always leads to theories, schools of thought and arguments that have opposing rivals, leading only to disagreement and conflict. In the acres of literature on philosophy, there is little in the way of definitive and insightful conclusions, and philosophical or theological differences have been responsible for many of the greatest conflicts in the history of humankind. Through meditation, our purpose is to reach that elusive state that allows us to relate all the conflicting arguments to a systematic hole. This is a difficult state to accomplish, but the benefits to the individual and our species of gaining insight on the relationship between mind and body make it a quest that would be worth the challenge.

It is worth noting that the conflicts between Western philosophical standpoints on the mind-body relationship are also present in yoga.

There are yoga traditions which emphases the bodily system over the mental one, and vice versa.

The Breath and the Mind

Neither of the opposing schools of thought need occupy much of our time; they are merely viewpoints, which are but one side of a complete whole and too limited for us to dwell on. In medical science and psychology, it is accepted that mental illness can be damaging to bodily functions, and physical injury or illness can affect the mind. We are psychophysical organisms, not merely bodies or disembodied minds. Hence in meditation, practitioners seek to explore the relationship between the breath – one of the body's most fundamental necessities – and the mind. This exploration should consist not of observations about the external manifestations they produce, but in the intrinsic relationship they share. Yoga teaches us that it is the spirit – a force of life or soul – that implements and regulates the min-body relationship. We have a spirit which is separate from both the mind and the body.

This is a key element of meditative practice, but the difficulty is that to define the spirit is an incredibly challenging task. We are some abstract, immaterial entity that expresses itself as a unification between thought and physical action. This is why when one of these two aspects is touched, so is the other – such is there unity by way of the spirit. This is why, in the meditation practice called pranayama, students are taught to focus the mind, and why doing so causes the breath to cease. One acts upon the other, and at close observation it is realised that the two are inseparable.

Any attempt at achieving harmony in the breathing process is beneficial. It is not necessary to focus to extremes on a certain technique to achieve only the harmonisation of breath as this is only one element of pure meditation. There are grammarians of the ancient Sanskrit language who study grammar throughout their entire lives without ever actually learning the literature. Similarly, practicing pranayama alone would be a mistake because it is not an end in itself; it is a part of the whole discipline that is meditation. All the limbs of meditation must be exercised and practiced to work together in a concentrated focus, because meditating is the total effort of a complex system of mind-body-spirit being focused into a singular concentrated energy.

It is often said that the limbs of meditation are akin to the rungs of a ladder, but this is a misleading analogy. As we travail the rungs of a ladder, we lose contact with the rungs we have climbed beyond, but in the limbs of yoga we must be in touch with them all at the same time. All the limbs are organically related and dependent upon one another so that, in an act of focused attention or concentration, they all take part at once. The 'self', in its entirety, practices meditation without the judgment of one limb as superior to another. The body-mind-spirit distinction is only really an expression to ease the understanding of an organism's totality; there is no definitive order in which they should be arranged, nor does the distinction have any meaning to the elements in themselves.

Chapter 2 – Finding the Sweet Spot

When a person begins the practice of meditation for the first time, they may feel overwhelmed by the new concepts they are bombarded with, as well as the elusiveness of the goals they have set. The notion of this 'sweet spot' or 'balance point' is one that can seem overwhelming in its unfamiliarity and elusive in its lack of specificity. It can seem like the only way you'll find it is by chancing upon it, as every time you feel you are closing in on what might be truly focused attention, it slips away. All that you need to know is that with practice, and without setting such goals for yourself, you will find that ease and consistency come naturally to you.

You will reach what some call the 'sweet spot' in your own way, and come to comprehend its meaning in a transcendent way that mere words cannot describe. Those who attempt to put it into words say that it is a point you reach mentally that allows you to balance two opposing states that are commonly experienced in meditation. On one side, there is the active exertion of trying to concentrate the mind, resist distractive thoughts and find the elusive state of mind that constitutes focused attention – all actions which can become crowded with frustrations, disappointments and judgments that ultimately restrict your ability to succeed. On the other side, there is essentially a state of sleep; extreme relaxation where you check out altogether from the experience and enter a subconscious state.

The 'sweet spot' is somewhere between these two, wherein you are able to focus the mind without having to try too hard, and relax it without allowing that focus to slip. It is here that we will be able to begin experiencing the benefits of meditations and filtering out the unnecessary baggage which clouds the spirit and becomes detrimental to both mind and body. At the sweet spot, the practitioner achieves maximum alertness and attentiveness without undue exertion, and simultaneously reaches a state of rest and relaxation without slipping out of touch. This is the balanced position that every practitioner aims to reach in order to progress their meditation to advanced levels.

The question, then, is simple: how do you gain access to this perfectly poised state amid the pull from the opposing forces that cloud your mind? The key is in your ability to exist only in the present moment. This is not a self-explanatory concept. We almost never exist only in the present moment – we are constantly processing what we see now in order to predict what will happen in the near future, often drawing on past experiences to find out how we should relate to what is happening or about to happen. We worry about what is to come, and dwell on what has passed. The truth is, the average person almost never allows him/herself to exist only in the present moment. But, if we wish to achieve the restful alertness of the 'sweet spot' in meditation, that is precisely what we must do. Without effort or complexity, you must live only in the moment at any one time. Simple, right?

Well, the present moment is like a doorway of opportunity that is ever-present from one moment to the next, if only we are able to filter out all distractions and give it our full attention. We always know that it is there, and stand in front of it constantly, but the chaos that surrounds it prevents us from seeing what it truly offers us. But what this doorway contains, what lies within the present moment at any point in time, is what is of most value to the individual. A person might say, and even believe, that they are present in the moment, but what are they present to? If it is only to their ceaseless thoughts and emotions, and the continuously changing aspects of life, this is not the presence that will yield the great benefits we seek from meditation.

We seek the hidden content of the present moment; some 'space' between thoughts and emotions. Through meditation, we practice turning our attention to that doorway of the present, allowing ourselves to become a completely self-contained entity and reaching that state not through force and relentless effort, but gently and effortlessly. Every moment that is 'the present' contains an infinity of stillness to explore, wherein the doorway is entered and its contents activated. The present becomes an eternal moment for you, as you simply experience what is, without judgment or expectation. Although this may seem like a vague description of some abstract nonsense, it is actually a very simple logical state of affairs. Without ever thinking about the past or the future, you become at one with the present moment as it moves from the former to the latter. You are still, yet moving through a self-regulating continuum, and the peace you experience by focusing entirely on that present is unlike any other, accepting your chaotic surroundings only as they pass by your connection with the present, without the need for them to instigate a thought. You are not cleansed of any mental or physical activity at all; rather, you focus your entirety on one thing.

It is far more difficult to put this into practice than it is to say it. The following is a list of 5 useful tips that will help you to overcome some of the common obstructions to finding your sweet spot and being present during your meditation practice.

Find your meditation space

It is important that you meditate in a private space free from any external disturbances. You should be able to feel safe, comfortable and completely at peace in your meditation space. If you have a bedroom to yourself, this is typically the simplest location for meditating, but if you would prefer a different location make sure it meets the requirements. Make sure that the spot in which you are going to meditate is clear and clean, without any clutter lying around. You need to create the perfect space for your practice.

Some people like to include in their meditation space some extra things that assist their practice. This might be a way to play some soothing meditation music, or some candles, or perhaps a diffuser for aromatherapy. Some people like to use a gong, and some enjoy the presence of certain flowers or crystals. Never underestimate the importance of making your meditation space perfect for you; this is the foundation of your practice.

Choose a comfortable sitting position

There are a number of recommended sitting positions to adopt during meditation; so much so, in fact, that it can become an unnecessary stress trying to ensure you are executing a position correctly! While the intentions of each instructed method are undeniably good, you may find that it is simpler for you to just sit in whatever way makes you feel comfortable. And this is perfectly fine! It is not true that unless you are seated in a specific position, you are not really meditating. You can sit cross-legged, or in a chair; whatever is comfortable and easy for you. The only necessity is that you sit upright to facilitate the flow of energy. Other than that, you are free to choose your own sitting position!

Clear your mind

Everybody has their own ways of doing this. The stretching movements of yoga, often followed by a shavasana, can facilitate this; stretching the muscles to loosen yourself up is a great way to facilitate this step of your practice. Also think about breathing deeply and slowly as you prepare to begin your meditation.

Merely sit and observe

This is what the preceding stages have been building up to. Once you begin your meditation, your task is to sit and observe the inner dialogue that plays out in your mind. What do you feel? What thoughts arise? Just observe and experience your inner workings without engaging them.

To force yourself to block out thoughts is to engage with a thought that will corrupt your practice. What you must instead do is allow thoughts to pass as you remain a passive observer; let your mind continue to move, but don't engage with its workings. It is as if you step outside of your own mind and watch it operate as if it were someone else's.

For example, the thought might pop into your head that you need to but some cereal for tomorrow. Observing this thought means that you are aware of its presence, and this is as far as you need to go. The mistake would be to allow yourself to react to that thought, perhaps with annoyance that you will have to visit the store to buy cereal, or an urgency that you must get to the store before it closes. These reactions mean you are engaging with the thought, and your meditation will be compromised if you allow this to happen.

One trick for detecting when your focus stumbles is to count slowly from 1 to 10, then return to 1 and continue repeating the process. When you feel your focus deviate, take note of what number you reached and you will have a rough idea of how long you were able to maintain your focus. This will gradually give you a way of measuring your progress while simultaneously occupying your mind to help strengthen that concentration. Bear in mind, though, that if you begin to think about beating your previous record as you approach it, you have already lost your focus!

The presence of your mind's thoughts during meditation means they are being cleared. They are elements of the chaos that is your mind, occasionally breaking through the multiplicity of thoughts screaming for attention inside your head to become the prominent thought at a given moment. Through the focus of meditation, they are being allowed to trickle away one by one. After repeated meditation practice for the long term, you will be able to reach that sought-after state of Zen-like mental quietness. This can only be found through quality meditation.

Your meditation sessions can last as long as you feel necessary. A good starting point would be 30 minutes, but in truth you can persist as long as you need to feel you have achieved the cleansing and refreshment you require. The longer a person meditates, particularly if they are able to sustain the requisite focus for long periods of time, the better.

Ending Your Meditation

When your meditation is finished, take your time returning to your normal physical state. Begin by acknowledging the physical reality around you, then your own physical body. Open your eyes slowly, begin to reawaken the limbs with small movements, and ease your way into physical activity. You might choose to reflect on your meditation before proceeding to go about your remaining business of the day; what thoughts, feelings and images did you experience? What peace did you enjoy? And what do you feel grateful for in the world?

Chapter 3 – Maintaining Open-Mindedness

If a friend told you that they stole $50 from a cash register at their local convenience store, what would you think? Would you lose respect for that friend, labelling them a thief? Perhaps you'd feel anger at the fact that you work hard to earn your money and this person simply takes money from someone else. Maybe you'd even feel some sense of pity for your friend, assuming they must have come upon hard times if they feel they must resort to stealing.

Well, how would it affect your judgment if they went on to tell you they took that money because they actually own the store, and they wanted to make a donation to a local orphanage?

A person whose mind is closed is often quick to jump to conclusions about what they see, hear or read. They pass judgment because they witness one part of a larger story and decide that what they have seen is 'good' or 'bad'; 'right' or 'wrong'. The first impression someone gets of a situation is too often the basis for their hasty conclusion. In reality, that first impression can often be incorrect, and allowing oneself to make decisions or judgments on that questionable basis can damage relationships, negatively affect health and alter one's perception of the world they live in.

Meditation can help us to develop a capacity to understand that things are not always as they seem. Opening your mind to a wider array of possibilities can have the following 8 positive effects on your life:

Your world is enriched. It is as a person who could only see in black and white being given the ability to recognize shades of colour. Your pallet cxpands as you acknowledge that there are far more than just 2 options for you to choose from. You can become liberated from the constraints of such limited possibilities, opening your eyes to the diversity the world has to offer.

You liberate your mind. Thinking you already have all the answers limits you from learning all that life has to offer. If you admit that there is much you do not know, you allow yourself the opportunity to explore new things and cross the boundaries that would otherwise have restricted your growth.

You can be open to change. Your thoughts and beliefs need to change before your actions and behaviours can. People who fail when they attempt to change what they perceive as 'negative' behaviours are the ones who attempt to do so without first changing the way they think. True change must occur from the inside out.

You have more fun. A willingness to try new, exciting things opens the door to a multitude of positive experiences! You can let go of whatever held you back in the past, opting to truly branch out and embrace life. The open minded will experiment with a wider range of things, and accrue a wealth of experiences along the way.

You will become better at solving problems. If you have a more developed ability to think outside the box, you become more effective in finding ways to solve all sorts of problems. You become adept at recognizing when certain methods and patterns are ineffective, and more creative in finding alternatives.

You have a greater capacity to love and be loved. When you transcend those passing judgments and hasty conclusions, you allow yourself to develop deeper connections with the people around you. You will give and receive love more openly because you are not so preoccupied with judging or being judged; you learn to accept people as they are.

You become more patient and tolerant. A greater sense of compassion and ability to empathise means you don't become so easily frustrated by others. You learn that, regardless of whether someone thinks a person is 'right' or 'wrong' to feel the way they do, the feelings that person is experiencing are valid and real for them.

You have more energy. When your mentality is not clouded with a preoccupation to figure everyone out and judge their behaviour, you are granted more mental energy to focus on positive things in life.

Loving-kindness meditation can be incorporated into your practice of focused-attention meditation to promote open-mindedness in your everyday life. Adding this to your practice can provide a perfect balance to the deeply introspective nature of focused-attention meditation, supporting you in bringing your meditation benefits into the world you live in.

There is no escaping the fact that we all live in a complex and challenging society, which burdens us with pressures and emotional stresses that can really plague the spirit. Unfortunately, most people do very little to develop the personal skills that can enable them to deal with these burdens. The salvation of a troubled mind is the capacity to find positivity in a cloud of negativity. Loving-kindness meditation is a Buddhist practice to develop one's capacity for selfless, or altruistic, love. Buddhist scripture states:

"Hatred cannot coexist with loving-kindness, and dissipates if supplanted with thoughts based on loving-kindness."

The practice of loving-kindness meditation brings about positive changes to attitude, systematically building a capacity for 'loving-acceptance'. It functions almost as a form of self-psychotherapy, enabling the practitioner to heal his/her own mind from its suffering. Through continued practice, you can experience the benefit of changing destructive thinking habits that lead to mental turmoil.

How is it done?

The first goal of practice is develop a 'loving acceptance' of yourself. Any resistance that a person encounters to their success in this type of meditation is rooted in some feeling of unworthiness regarding the self.

This is the first thing to be worked on, enabling a person to conquer self-doubt and negativity in order to form a basis upon which to build a love and compassion towards others.

Who are the people we aim to develop loving-kindness towards?

- A respected authority figure, such as a spiritual teacher, or 'guru'

- Someone of personal significance, such as a close friend or family member

- A neutral person, meaning somebody whom you know but have no emotional opinion of; an acquaintance

- A hostile person , meaning a rival or even an enemy

Beginning with the self, then systematically developing your loving-kindness towards the 4 people listed above, in the order of that list, is the process of loving-kindness meditation. This process will break down any barriers that restrict your interaction with the world around you, opening your mind to the multitude of perspectives that exist in any given situation. The breakdown of these mental divisions will eliminate the source of much of the mental turmoil you experience.

One word of caution: the person of 'personal significance' that you choose should not be someone for whom you could develop romantic or sexual attraction towards; lust is seen as a great obstacle to achieving loving-kindness.

Seek out the people who can fill the roles at each stage of the process; if a person doesn't work out in one of the roles, look elsewhere until you find someone that does.

Ways of arousing loving-kindness feelings

1. Visualisation — Generate a mental image; see yourself or the person you wish to direct the feeling towards smiling back at you, or just in a state of happiness.
2. Reflection — Think about the positive qualities the person has, or acts of benevolence they have done. Even towards yourself; make positive observations about yourself, as you see them.
3. Auditory — this is the most abstract, yet simple method. Repeating an internalized mantra can bring about inner peace and nurture feelings of loving-kindness.

These three techniques are devices to help the practitioner invoke feelings of loving-kindness. A practitioner can use all three, or focus their attention on just one or two of the methods; it really depends what works best for the individual. As the positive feelings begin to arise, you must switch your attention from the chosen method to the feeling itself, as this feeling is the primary objective of your practice. Keep the mind fixed on that feeling, returning to the techniques only if the mind deviates or the feelings begin to significantly weaken. Once a person can comfortably maintain the feeling without having to frequently return to one of the methods that create it, they are ready to progress to the next stage of their practice.

This second stage is called 'Directional Pervasion', in which you gradually attempt to project your loving-kindness in all directions around where you sit. To enhance one's ability to project in this way, they are encouraged to form mental connections with loving friends and like-minded communities in the world; by focusing the mind on these things whilst experiencing the loving-kindness feeling, we project it towards all that surrounds us.

As a person's practice matures, they will most likely find that, at some point, they experience a spontaneous event we call Non-Specific Pervasion. This is a moment of indiscriminate, unconditional love that emanates from your being and encapsulates everything in the universe! This experience is the manifestation of loving-kindness meditation at full maturation, in which specifically-targeted love is transcended, allowing the practitioner to feel the same love and compassion that is unattached to anything specific. It is unconditional, and it is universal.

Loving-kindness is a meditation that must be lived, and as such cannot be restricted to the abstracted formal ceremony of sitting practice. The positivity and love it inspires must be taken out into the world, reflecting in your interactions with elements of everyday life. Applying the practice to everyday life means showing compassion and friendliness, and having an open mind towards every person and ting you relate to, without judgment or discrimination.

The ways of achieving this state are numerous, as practices vary between different schools. This chapter serves to introduce you to the basic principles and techniques, giving you a foundation upon which to build as you study and learn for yourself, should you choose to do so. This practice is complementary to other meditative practices, and is one of the essential elements towards achieving the most elusive state of 'enlightenment'.

Chapter 4 - Meditation with Purpose

The concept of 'meditation' is defined by a number of meanings. It is for this reason that it can be so mystifying for those that attempt to engage with it and achieve its goals. The purest description of its meaning is that it is the way, or the journey, by which a person is led internally to a state of being consisting of calm awareness and keen intuition. It is therefore more accurate to understand meditation as a tool to help reach an ultimate objective, rather than an end in itself. This chapter advocates meditating with purpose, or meditating as a means to an end, to apply meditation as a holistic practice rather than fitting into a single category wherein meditation is the goal in itself.

It is common for the chanting of repetitious words or phrases, or a commitment to focus entirely on some external image, to be used in meditative practices as a means to assist a practitioner in their attempts to transcend the chaos of ordinary thought. These practices are usually deeply immersed in particular cultural traditions, and it can be argues that they constitute a number of principles that aren't really relevant to modern society. It is often argues that certain aspects of these traditions restrict them to merely scratching the surface in terms of spiritual experience, leaving the deepest of modern needs undiscovered and unresolved.

Of course, it can give some level of relief to be liberated from the relentless compulsions and distractions of uncontrolled thought and emotion, and traditional meditation techniques can provide this relief. But a true transcendence of mental chaos comes as a result of some kind of analysis of the content of our thoughts, so that psychological considerations can be incorporated into our practice, rather than teaching yourself to ignore thoughts and thus push what could be more troubling content into the unconscious mind. Many complexes, neuroses and problems may be present in the average person's mind, and the only way these can truly be addressed is by listening to the thoughts they cause. Don't be fooled into thinking that one can achieve a transcendental, detached existence by simply conditioning oneself to avoid or ignore thought; psychology teaches us that doing so will bury those thoughts in places where they will continue to pull on our minds and bodies.

In order for us to be liberated from their hold over us, we must learn to understand them for what they really are; a consequence of emotional and psychological needs and desires at every level of our being. There exists a constructive, healthy way of thinking, and its opposing, destructive alternative, and the true purpose of meditation must be to bring a practitioner to a profound understanding of that distinction between thought patterns.

Exploring the Subconscious Mind

A healthy mind, through its inherent comprehension of the distinction between healthy and unhealthy thinking, will be enabled to entertain thought as the origin of inspired inner direction and creativity. Thus, with the correct application of meditating with purpose, our practice encourages the capacity to possess a mind of the utmost discernment, with the aim of being able to make clear and correct decisions as to which thought patterns are worthy of support, and which need to be eliminated from the mind as they arise.

Furthermore, is must be understood that any form of meditation that purports to achieve swift results is likely to be a relatively superficial practice; achieving the depth of understanding that we uphold as the ultimate objective of meditation takes time and discipline. Meditation practice that is extremely challenging and slow to progress in the early stages is the type that will eventually lead to more profound results if a practitioner is able to persevere with it. There are no shortcuts in meditation, and any techniques that purport to offer them will never take you to the purest of conclusions.

The truth is, it is far easier to merely ignore the observation of thought content than it is to confront it directly. Once you have learned, through a meditative practice, some techniques for not engaging with thoughts, you will find it becomes increasingly easy to do so; proponents of meditation with purpose will say that this method of practice will never lead to the pure objective of self-renewal. They will state that in order to achieve a calm and centred state of existence, one must be prepared to direct their practice towards integrating the promotion of healthy thinking into their meditation, reserving the ability to not engage with thoughts only for when negative thought processes arise.

Learning to connect with, and understand, the subconscious mind takes time and dedication. In subconscious thought processes we can find all the forces and desires that play upon our conscious mind and motivate us to feel and act in the ways that we do. Facing this dimension of the mind forces us to confront our imperfections and inadequacies through an examination of the thoughts that act upon us from a level beneath our conscious awareness. These thoughts are alive, but largely undetected, until they find a way to surface in an emotion or desire that directs our conscious thoughts and actions.

Certain research groups have devised a method of identifying or detecting latent, subconscious thought derivations through the use of a device similar to the polygraph machine used in lie-detecting tests. The person undergoing the test is encouraged to look into their past in an attempt to discover memories which instigate a significant emotional response, identified by the 'biofeedback machine' registering the changes those emotions cause in certain body functions. Through this method, a person can discover unacknowledged past emotions that have been buried in the subconscious, providing the opportunity to explore them and draw conclusions about what affect they have on the subject's present thoughts and actions.

Once you are made increasingly conscious of powerful emotional affecters that have long been buried in the subconscious, you can work on purging your mind of the response patterns they have long exerted on your thought processes. Through this realization, the researchers believe, you can liberate yourself entirely of such dormant influences on your life, enabling you to truly move towards the tranquillity of mind that is the objective of meditative practice.

The Missing Link: Prevention

The one thing that would appear to be lacking in this research, however, is the development of a non-emotional capacity that relates to the discovery of dormant thoughts to ensure the destructive thought patterns won't resurface in future. It is here that meditation really comes into its own; as the phase of discovering sources of mental chaos and trauma is complete, so begins the process of preparing the mind for its inevitable future encounters with similar emotional programming taking place. Through meditation we can conquer the mental chaos that already exists, and condition the mind to prevent similar chaos arising as a result of future experiences.

Through personal, private meditation, a person can perform this 'self-audit' on their own mind. Additionally, one can also take the necessary steps to be prepared for future experiences that could lead to new subconscious thoughts causing problems. This does not mean that the person becomes cold and emotionless to the point that they become unable to experience the highs and lows of a rich and varied life. It means, rather, that the thoughts and emotions are monitored and assessed by a higher awareness, strengthened continuously by dedication to daily meditation practice. By slowing and considering the onset of emotional reactions, the practitioner begins to gain a profound comprehension of the fact that he or she has the opportunity to make a choice between interpretations of all experiences. One can choose to react emotionally and thereby allow a foundation for negative thinking, or one can withhold powerful emotional judgments in favour of dispassionate observation of the fallibility of other people without allowing it to consume their mind.

It is a great power to be in control of your emotional responses; one which brings a person to a higher consciousness wherein they can experience life in a way that was previously blocked from their awareness and understanding. The doors of perception and creativity become fully open, allowing the ultimate seizure of opportunities and understanding of situations, and thus the ability to fulfil the true extent of one's potential. A person's inner reality will flourish under these circumstances.

In Summary...

The buried, negative, traumatic memories seep into your being and obstruct the path of true growth as a person. To overcome this, one must identify and unlock those deep-rooted emotional thought triggers from the unconscious and process them, and then train the mind to be able to avoid taking on similar destructive baggage in the future. This takes time and dedication, but can set a person on the true path towards fulfilling their potential as a human being.

Meditation is an active practice, and it should not be considered an end in itself; it is merely a tool for a person to achieve their goals of personal and spiritual development, eventually allowing them to reach a state of love, light and peaceful awareness and intuition.

Meditation, as a practice, can be defined in several ways; it can be to engage in deep contemplation or reflection, or it can be a mental exercise to heighten one's spiritual awareness. It is sometimes associated with Buddhism or Hinduism, while many consider it a purely secular activity. Contemplative practices are also prominent in Judeo-Christian culture, wherein significant figures have been known to 'meditate' as a form of reflecting on some lessons learned.

The suggestion is that meditation should not be considered to be a process of merely emptying the mind of thoughts altogether, it should instead be a practice of consciously discerning between thoughts that are harmful or beneficial, and processing/expelling the negative so as to fill the mind and spirit with all that is good and positive. This can bring about a real feeling of release during meditative practice, where you no longer have to exert such effort to cleanse yourself of thought altogether.

Typical mental chatter, however, such as how you should answer a tricky question in an email or whether you should be folding your laundry, are the clutter that needs to be eliminated during meditation. How can we move beyond this troublesome fog in order to gain access to a higher mental perspective that encapsulates the mental considerations that truly matter? Here are some suggestions for meditation with purpose:

1. Silently ask yourself a really significant question

Simply propelling our minds to consider really big questions can set the benchmark for the trajectory of our thoughts. Questions like "where does the universe end, and where does it begin?" or "if the universe was started by a big bang, what caused the big bang?" These thoughts can connect you with the higher planes of thinking, and taking the time to grasp the concepts they are attached to can be a great way to initiate your practice.

As some insights begin to dawn in your mind, your thought happens will be transformed for that period. This can bring about a profound stillness, and a release of concern about the worries that trouble you as you become more aware of their minute significance to the grand picture of the universe.

2. Consider the idea that you're a part of creation, or Divinity

We all experience those moments when we are overawed by the wondrous sights and sounds of creation; like when you are away from the city and catch a moment where you look up at the night sky and witness the universe in all its glory. The sense of wonder at the vastness of creation is matched only by the beauty of knowing that everything is connected. Objects that are thousands of light years away are presenting themselves to you, blessing you with their light to show that time and space are but dimensions of a whole that we are a part of. This connectedness of all creation is seen by many as the presence of Divinity.

When you experience such moments, you activate the part of you that recognizes its share in the spiritual unity of everything that exists. This contemplation of being connected to everything in the universe can help you gain access to the state of mind necessary to engage in a practice of successful meditation.

3. **Absorb those ideas, and bask in the insights they bring**

   Whichever option you choose to activate your higher thought processes, allow the new insights and realizations to settle in place of old ways of thinking. The humility that can sweep over you when you contemplate those big questions has a tremendous calming effect, nullifying the prominence of trivial concerns. Humility also allows you to empathize better, and see situations from a greater number of perspectives. The mental space and openness makes it easier to allow fresh insights to settle into the mind and be brought forward into subsequent activities.

In order to experience the benefits of these wider perspectives, you need to take the time to refresh the new thinking patterns frequently by repeating the techniques described above regularly.

Chapter 5 – Guided Meditations

As previously alluded to, the stress and pressure of living in the modern world are leading to an increase in the popularity of meditation. People are becoming increasingly interested in finding new ways to relax, de-stress and connect with a spiritual dimension of themselves to make more sense of the chaos they experience in their day-to-day lives.

To cater for this increase in popularity, and to make meditation more accessible for beginners, there has been a surge in the prominence of guided meditation classes. This is one of the easiest ways for beginners to learn how meditation works, and practice their own technique which they could later apply in a private setting. If you are thinking about incorporating meditation into your life, but don't know where to begin, guided meditation may be just the answer you're looking for.

Guided Meditation takes the Pressure off you

Meditation is not only great for health, but when you are experiencing effective practices and the results it yields, it is incredibly enjoyable and inspiring as it carries you towards the inner peace you crave. Guided meditation is, simply put, the easiest way to meditate with the reassurance that you're getting it right!

Traditional, unguided meditation practices require some real effort on your part, and can feel like a shot in the dark when you start out. This can make it more stressful and time consuming, with little gain in the early stages that could soon put you off the practice altogether. Through guided meditation, you are helped every step of the way through the mental processes of clearing the mind and achieving stillness and presence. Your guide will literally walk you through the process from beginning to end.

What could be more effortless and relaxing than listening to soothing, tranquil music whilst you are guided into a state of deep meditation?

In its ease of access, guided meditation can be a very powerful tool for achieving the personal development results meditation has to offer.

The Power of Guided Meditation

Guided meditations tend to differ from traditional meditation in that they utilize the power of your imagination to direct your mind to the state it requires for effective meditation. Your own capacity for visualization is honed, transforming your mentality to one that can bring about genuine personal change, and many practitioners claim this makes guided meditation even more potent than passive meditation.

Creative visualization is defined as the use of harnessing of mental imagery to bring about positive change in one's mentality. Such visualization techniques are now commonly used for motivation and positive psychiatry in such diverse fields as business, arts, sports, religion, alternative medicine, psychotherapy and self-improvement. The underlying principle is that the mind is unable to discern between an event that actually takes place, and one that was vividly imagines. Think about it; have you ever had a really vivid dream that leaves you unable to recall whether something actually happened or was just something you dreamt? When this occurs, we often find ourselves only able to make the distinction by finding some empirical evidence that shows whether that memory was of something real or imagined. And even then, the emotion that the dream caused can linger on the mind.

Guided meditations lead you to vividly imagine positive experiences that are carefully crafted to represent, either literally or symbolically, the positive changes you wish to bring about in your life.

The environment and atmosphere that is created for guided meditation is one of deep relaxation; it is important to achieve this state to allow the imagination to concoct the most powerful visualizations possible. You become immersed in the aura of the guided practice, listening to soothing, positive instructions while basking in the holistic experience of the environment that has been created. As a result, you will experience immediate benefits from even a single practice! You'll feel better physically, emotionally, spiritually and mentally.

Of course, these are only short term benefits and, in meditation terms, relatively superficial. Guided meditations are flexible so that they can be tailored to meet the diverse goals of a multitude of individuals who wish to engage in it. The outcomes that different forms of guided meditation are said to yield include:

Improving clarity in life

Enhancing creativity

Treating depression

Increasing confidence and personal empowerment

Emotional and physical healing

Profoundly deep relaxation

Opening the heart and healing relationships

Spiritual development

Improving performance in business or sports

Experiencing expanded awareness

If guided meditation is well crafted, it will include positive suggestions and visualizations that lead your mind to a state wherein the goals you set out with can be realized. Making the mental, emotional and spiritual changes your life needs is an incredibly important task; if you remain hampered by destructive attributes that have become embedded in your being, you will never be able to overcome the barriers that obstruct you on the path to reaching your full potential as a human being.

Meditation is the answer, and guided meditation is a fantastic place to start, easing your access to meditative techniques and carrying you to a state of mental stillness, in which your mind can be cleared of the relentless chatter and clutter of unwanted and trivial thoughts. This creates the space to flood your mentality with visualization experiences that effect positive change.

A guided meditation that it specifically tailored to your needs may also make use of very carefully crafted symbolism that can potently connect with the deepest levels of your subconscious, or even unconscious, mind. The deeper levels of the mind often surface in bizarre, abstract imagery – just think of one of your more peculiar dreams – so connecting with it in a similar way can bring about more profound healing if it strikes the right chord.

In Summary...

Guided meditation is more than just a relaxing social experience that helps cope with stress; it can actually help practitioners experience the benefits of traditional meditation in an accessible, personally-tailored way. By making meditation more accessible, guided practice allows beginners to engage in deep meditation without the pressure of having to figure out the intricacies by themselves. It immerses you in an environment that promotes profound relaxation and stillness, easing the process of achieving mental focus and spiritual presence, then walks you through a series of visualizations that harness the power of the imagination to bring about the insights and perceptions needed to enact positive change. You could definitely do worse than giving guided meditation a shot, particularly if you are a beginner who feels overwhelmed at the challenge of successfully engaging in meditation.

Chapter 6 - Meditation in Everyday Life

Throughout the course of their training, practice and eventual attainment of the status of master, a pianist will continuously play scales. The finest concert pianists will continue practicing scales as they prepare for a performance; it is a fundamental practice that ensures every aspect of their playing remains in peak condition.

Every tennis player continues to practice their swing. It's the first thing a beginner must learn, as it is fundamental to performing any type of shot with the required measure of control. Every match begins with a 'knock up' to get the swing functioning for the match ahead. Basic skills must always be kept sharp.

Seated, private meditation is the fundamental practice that a meditator continues to maintain his or her fundamental skills. The meditator's craft is that of experiencing and living their own life, and the tool is the set of sensory apparatus the body is equipped with. Even the greatest masters of meditation must continue to practice seated meditation, because it serves to maintain sharpness in the fundamental skills required enact their craft. The important lesson here is this: seated meditation is not, in itself, the craft of the meditator; it is merely the fundamental practice that must be continuously enacted to sharpen the tools which enable the craftsman to exist and experience in the 'right' way. Meditation that is not applied to daily life is empty and superficial.

The deepest purpose of meditation is no less than the complete and permanent transformation of one's sensory and cognitive experience. In other words, it is enlightenment; a revolutionary change to the way you experience life. Periods of seated practice are the time we set aside to generate new mental habits that we can apply to daily life. We learn new ways to receive and interpret sensory information. We develop new methods of processing conscious thought, and new approaches to cope with the range of emotions that can wash over us throughout our activities. The new mental behaviours we develop through seated practice are to be carried over into every other part of our lives; otherwise meditation is a fruitless practice, like some abstract or theoretical game that merely distracts us from the difficulties of our existence rather than teaching us to deal with them. It is essential that we make the required effort to connect what we learn through meditation to every other segment of our lives. A certain amount will naturally carry over, but this process alone will be slow and uncontrolled. Without taking a holistic approach to meditation, you are likely to find yourself feeling that it is leading nowhere, and eventually lose interest in continuing your practice.

One of the most unforgettable moments as you progress through the practice of meditation is the realization that you are actually meditating whilst undertaking some unrelated daily activity. You might be driving to work, or watering the garden, and it just spontaneously comes into being. This is your first glimpse of what true meditation means; you are struck with the possibility that the transcendent state of consciousness could become a permanent feature of your life, and you are instilled with a joy and motivation unlike anything you have felt before. It becomes clear to you that there is a realistic possibility that the remainder of your days could be spent in a state of liberation from the chaos, fears and trivial chatter that so clouds the mind of the average person. As stated, it's an unforgettable moment; an epiphany.

Fulfilling that vision, however, becomes a case of actively working to carry over the discoveries you make from your practice into the rest of your world. Think of the moment you stand and exit your practice as the most important moment of it – you can then choose to leave the meditation behind and carry on as normal, or carry the skills on into every move you make until your next practice.

It is crucial to gain an inherent comprehension of what meditation truly is. It is not some special posture, or a specific mantra or even a set of mental exercises. It is a holistic activity to cultivate mindfulness, and the application of said mindfulness once it has been developed. You do not necessarily have to be sitting to meditate; it can be done while washing the dishes, taking a shower, riding a bike or typing an e-mail. The presence and awareness of meditative practice must be enacted in every aspect of life. This is very difficult to do.

It is through practice in a seated posture, in an environment of peace and isolation, that we cultivate awareness because these are the ideal circumstances for doing so; it makes it easier. Meditation while in motion is a far more advanced skill. In the midst of crowds and noise, it becomes even more challenging! But the ultimate challenge is in maintaining a meditative state when in a situation that would usually illicit vast amounts of emotions; on romantic occasions, or during heated arguments, for example. To the beginner, quiet practice is likely to be the only way to reach the required state of consciousness for practice.

Nevertheless, the ultimate goal of practice is to build one's focus, awareness and presence to such a level that it is able to remain unshaken in the midst of anything the world can throw at it. Life offers a great number of challenges daily, and the dedicated meditator is rarely bored.

Carrying your meditation into daily life is not a simplistic process; you only have to try it to see this for yourself. The transition from your seated meditation back into 'real life' is, for the majority of practitioners, a significant leap. It is all too easy for the focus and tranquillity to dissipate as the world crashes back down upon you with its pressures and stresses, and it can feel like the meditation practice has left us no better off than before. Through the millennia that meditation has existed, practitioners have developed a number of exercises aimed at narrowing the gap between the meditation and the 'real world'. The following techniques are designed to help you take the skills gained in seated practice with you as you transition back into daily activities:

1. Walking Meditation

Everyday life is filled with motion and activity. Sitting in complete stillness, without noise or disturbance, is simply not something that occurs in the average experience of modern society. Thus, when we transition from seated practice to daily life, the calmness and focus we gained is driven out of us as the activity of the day becomes prominent. Some transitional exercise is needed to teach us the skill of retaining that stillness in the midst of so much motion. 'Walking meditation' eases that very transition from static contemplation to daily motion; it's meditation while moving, and is commonly used as an alternative to seated practice. Walking is particularly useful at times when we feel frustrated or restless, as it can help to dissipate that anxious energy that might otherwise interfere with the contemplative practice during seated meditation. It can therefore be a way to prepare for the seated version as well as an alternative to it.

Traditional Buddhist practice consists of frequent retreats into isolation to engage in standard sitting meditation; these retreats are often for significant lengths of time that is devoted exclusively to practice, and takes place in a monastery where no other commitments are required of the practitioner – a monk may spend weeks, months or even years meditating in this way! This dedication is all-consuming and extremely demanding on the mind and body, and without an already-vast experience of meditation can be counter-productive in an effort to achieve the meditative goals. Think about it: sitting still for ten hours at a time will cause pain and stiffness in the average person that would far exceed any presence and stillness that might be attained through the meditative practice. A beneficial retreat, therefore, would generally consist of seated meditation interspersed with walking meditation at regular intervals, with short breaks in between to ease the strain on the mind.

To enact walking meditation, you first need to find a private place in which there is sufficient space for you to walk at least five to ten paces in one direction. You will be pacing back and forth very slowly, and will appear to the outsider to look odd and disconnected from your surroundings. Performing this practice on your front lawn will bring with it the unnecessary distraction of curious onlookers, so you are best off choosing a private place.

The physical instructions are not complicated: select an unobstructed area and start at one end; stand for a minute or so in an attentive posture, holding your arms in whatever position feels comfortable for you; on an inhale, lift the heel of one foot, then rest that foot on its toes as you exhale; next, while inhaling, lift that foot and carry it forward to touch the ground as you exhale. Repeat this process for each foot until you reach the end of your space, then turn and repeat the entire process. Every action should be performed very slowly. Your head should be upright and relaxed, with your eyes open but not focused on anything in particular. Pay no attention to your surroundings, as they are merely distractions and not relevant to your practice. Be aware of any tensions that arise in the body, and make sure they are released as soon as they are detected. It is not important to look graceful or elegant; this is not an athletic exercise or a dance! It is an exercise in mental presence and awareness; your aim is to achieve total alertness and focus upon the unjudged, uninterrupted experience of walking. Focus your entire attention upon the sensations coming from the feet and legs registering as much objective information as possible as each foot moves. Be submerged entirely in the pure sensation of the motion, such that you are aware of every subtle nuance and intricacy of the body's movements. Every change in tactile sensation must be registered, and every muscular pull and release acknowledged.

It will become apparent to you, if your focus is sufficient, that each seemingly fluid motion is actually a series of small, jerky movements. Don't miss this observation; in order to maximize your sensitivity in the present moment, it can help to break down larger movements into the tiny motions that constitute it. Each foot is subjected to a roll forward, a lift, a swing and a grounding motion, and each of these stages has its own beginning, middle and end. To attune yourself entirely to these motions, try to take mental notes of the passing of every stage. Doing so will familiarize you with the intricate series of movements, making sure none go unnoticed. As your awareness of the myriad details involved in every movement, you will have no time for forming words or unrelated thoughts; you will be totally immersed in your awareness of your own sensations. The feet and legs will become your entire universe! If your mind wanders, adhere to the usual principle of not engaging with the thought, and return your focus to the task at hand. Don't look at your feet and legs during this process, and don't attempt to construct a mental picture of what they are doing. As the great Bruce Lee once said: "Don't think. Feel!" Concepts and images such as feet and legs are irrelevant; all that is needed are the sensations that flow through your being. You may find, as a beginner, that you experience some issues with balance, but with time you will familiarize your body with the movements and they will become easier. If frustration arises, note its presence and let it go.

The intention of this walking meditation practice is that it floods your consciousness with simple sensations that you can focus your entire attention on, pushing all other thought out of the mind. There is no room for thought, judgment or emotion, nor for visualizing or breaking the activity down into a series of concepts. There is only a continuous flow of tactile and kinaesthetic sensation; a cyclical flood of raw experience. This is an escape into reality, not an escape from it. Whatever insights come to us during this practice are directly applicable to all other aspects of our active, motion-filled days.

2. Postures

We must always uphold, as the goal of our practice, the state of being fully aware of every aspect of our experience of the present moment with each passing second. Much of what are bodies do and experience takes place unconsciously, that is without our awareness or intervention, but the mind is another matter. We pass a significant amount of our time lost in a fog of daydreams and passing thoughts, as if they are running on autopilot.

This imbalance is something we must seek to address; rather than allowing the musings of the mind to continue in their dominance of our attention from one moment to the next, we should seek to recognize the kinaesthetic and tactile sensations that continuously interact with our bodies. Every one of those sensations is barraging the brain with data incessantly, but we seem to switch off the part of our consciousness that interacts with that data, allowing it to pour only into the lower levels of the mind and never feature in our awareness. Buddhists have developed an exercise that opens the floodgates and lets this data pour into our consciousness; it's a technique to make some part of the unconscious, conscious!

Your body is contorted into all manner of shapes and postures in any given day; you sit and stand, walk and lie down, bend, crawl, run and sprawl, all in the time between waking up and going back to bed! Students of meditation are urged to continuously remain aware of this ever-changing dance of activity. Every few minutes throughout each day, take a few seconds to acknowledge the posture of your body. Don't do so in a way to make any kind of judgment on what you observe, as this is not an exercise in correcting posture or attempting to look a certain way for some external purpose. Simply sweep your attention down through each area of your body, feeling the sensations that are present in the way you carry it at that moment. Silently note the posture so that your awareness o the body remains ever-present. This may sound ridiculously simplistic, but that makes it no less significant. With the necessary commitment, this is a powerful exercise in maintaining an awareness of your present sensations that can revolutionize your experience of daily activities. You will tap into an entirely new dimension of the senses, as would a blind man whose sight has been restored.

3. Slow-Motion Action

As previously noted, every action you make is actually a series of separate components. For example, the simple process of tying your shoelace can be broken down into a system of subtle body movements. For the average person, the vast majority of these movements pass by unobserved. To promote the overriding habit of continuous mindfulness, you can resolve to carry out simple activities at a very low speed; this enables you to carefully observe every nuance of the action.

Sitting at a table and drinking a cup of coffee is one time you could enact this exercise. There is a great deal of experience that takes place here. Observe your posture as you sit, and feel the handle of the cup between your fingers. Smell the coffee's unique aroma, and feel the heat of the cup, the motion of your arm as it lifts the cup to your mouth, and the taste of the coffee as it first hits your tongue. The keep your focus on the reverse of the actions that raised the cup, and the way your arm perhaps contacts the table as you place the cup down. The entire process is something that is usually taken for granted, but is actually an intricate process with symbiotic relationships between sensations that are unified in an overall experience. Paying full attention to the process opens your eyes to its beauty, and your mindfulness is amplified by your detached sensation to the slow-motion execution of every stage of the coffee drinking activity.

This same approach can be made with a number of daily activities. Intentionally slowing your actions, words and thoughts enables you to dwell far more deeply on every aspect of those processes, and with full attentiveness you can make some astonishing discoveries. When this technique is first adopted, it can be challenging to maintain this deliberate pace during most activities, but the skill to do so grows through practice. It can occur that the profound realizations made during seated meditation pale in comparison with those that take place as we focus our attention to our inner workings during activity. In this environment, we are truly able to observe the mechanisms that are our emotions and passions, and thus gauge the reliability of our reasoning and the necessity of our responses in any number of situations. In this way, we can chip away at the pretences and destructive responses that we maintain as we interact with our surroundings.

It will be the case that much of these insights are surprising, some of them even disturbing or difficult to accept, but all will be useful. Through the purity of present attention we bring order to the clutter that gather in the recesses of the mind. As you begin meeting the challenge of maintaining such clear comprehension in the midst of life's constant motion and activity, you gain the ability to remain objective, rational and peaceful while discerning between what is useful to the mind and what would ultimately add to the trivial clutter that clouds the average person's consciousness. You will eventually have the epiphany that the disorganized nature of your mind was largely responsible for much of your own mental suffering; misery, fear and anxiety are self-generated, and as your comprehension of these mental processes grows, the hold they have on you will dissipate.

4. Breath Coordination

In seated meditation, the primary focus is on the breath. Complete focus upon the ever changing cycle of breath keeps us firmly grounded in the present moment. This same principle can be carried over to times of movement; you can co-ordinate any given activity with the rhythm of your breathing. This will lend a fluidity to your movements while smoothing out many of the abrupt transitions. Activity therefore becomes easier to focus on, creating the mindful presence necessary for meditation. Ideally, meditation should be a 24-7 practice, and this is a highly practical way to implement this.

The state of mindfulness is one of mental readiness; the mind is never burdened with preoccupations or bound in concern about the future. Whatever challenges or considerations arise are dealt with instantly. When this state of mindfulness is achieved, even the nervous system is infused with a freshness and resilience that promotes insight. No problem poses anything more than a momentary concern before being dealt with swiftly and efficiently. When the rare circumstances arise where no solution seems possible, the mind doesn't buckle under the weight of worries and fear. The well-honed intuition becomes a very practical characteristic in daily life.

5. Stolen Moments

For the dedicated practitioner of meditation, there is no such thing as wasted time. The moments in a day where there is nothing to do can be capitalized on by being used for meditation. This means that any space of time in your day can become constructive; while waiting anxiously for a doctor's appointment, meditate on that anxiety. While queuing at the post office, meditate on your impatience or frustration. Keep alert to your inner workings throughout the day, being mindful of all that is taking place at any given moment, even if it is just the time elapsing between important events. Capitalize on moments of quiet and solitude, just as you take advantage of activities that require little or no active thought to complete. Every moment is valuable to your practice, so you should never feel that time has been 'wasted'.

6. Concentration on all Activities

Your ultimate goal in meditation in everyday life is to maintain that presence of mind through every activity and perception that passes throughout the day. This should start the moment you awaken, and cease the moment you fall asleep. This is an incredibly challenging task to set yourself all in one go, so you should not expect to be able to achieve it in the short term. Work at it step by step, with a commitment and belief in its value, and your abilities will grow over time. Just as it has been suggested that you break each motion down into its sections, you should try doing the same to your days. Plan to dedicate regular intervals of time each day to being mindful, trying to make those moments coincide with activities like washing, dressing, eating and so forth; activities that you can perform without extensive concentration, allowing you to focus on presence and mindfulness whilst you engage in them. Think also about observing the range of mental states that you encounter: pleasant or unpleasant feeling; those which you are indifferent to; hindrances or feelings of sympathy and empathy. The routine is up to you, but keep in mind the idea of continuously spotting various inner workings, and preserving that mindfulness as fully as possible throughout the day.

Eventually you want to have a daily routine wherein there is as little difference as possible between your mental state during meditation, and that of all other daily experience. The two should naturally, and eventually effortlessly, slide together, such that the almost continuous motion of your body is constantly observed internally. And even when there is not motion, there is breathing. And as the activity of the mind persists, you will learn to remain an impartial observer to all that transpires therein. Through the dedicated application of meditation, you will never be at a loss for inner workings worthy of your attentiveness or awareness.

To attain the highest levels of consciousness, your practice must be applied to everyday life. The trials and tribulations of the world are what challenge you to maximize your discipline and commitment, acting as a fire that purifies your self-destructive mental habits and practices, offering insights as you observe with objectivity the trappings of your own mind. If it is the case that your meditation is having no beneficial effect on your everyday conflicts and challenges, then it simply isn't working. If your insights about yourself and the way you relate to your surroundings are not becoming clearer, then your meditation is too superficial. Without attempting to apply your practice to everyday life, you can't know if it is offering you the benefits it should be.

Mindfulness is a universal practice; not something you can pick up and drop at your convenience. It is holistic, and you do it all the time. Successful meditation comes into its own only when you descend from your fortress of solitude, and if it only seems to benefit you while you are in hiding then it is still underdeveloped. The meditator learns that attention can be perpetually paid to the birth, evolution and decay of all physical, mental and spiritual phenomena in the context of the present moment. Nothing is ignored, and nothing is expelled; all is observed and acknowledged continuously as it passes by in an endless process of change.

If you find yourself bored, then meditate on your boredom; observe how it feels, how it acts upon your mind, and what it is composed of. If you are angry, do the same thing for that anger. Any feelings or emotions you experience have mechanics that can be explored, and you must investigate them rather than attempt to flee from them. If you are gripped by a dark depression, explore this powerful emotion in a detached and honest way, exploring the labyrinth of your mind and charting its routes. That way you will be better prepared to deal with that depression when it returns in the future.

Meditating your way through the ups and downs of life is intensely rigorous and challenging, but through dedicated persistence it leads to a state of mental flexibility and resilience that is without equal. A true practitioner will keep the mind open at all times, maintaining a curiosity to explore and investigate every experience that is encountered, in a detached and objective way. This way, one becomes a conduit for truth as it emanates from any source at any time. This state of consciousness is what is required to achieve liberation, or 'enlightenment'.

It is said that enlightenment may be attained spontaneously and unexpectedly if the mind is kept in a state of meditative readiness. The tiniest, most arbitrary of perceptions could be the catalyst that propels the consciousness into that state; it is said that the perception itself is not important, rather it is in the way one attends to that perception. If you are ready, it could happen to you as you read this sentence! It could be the sound of these words in your head, or the appearance of the letters before your eyes. Enlightenment is not something that can be planned for, it happens when it does.

Final Thoughts

Meditation is a practice that all manner of people will take an interest in for just as great a number of reasons. As an ancient practice of Eastern culture seeped in tradition and notions of spiritual enrichment, it is intended to be a means to attain a transcendent state of consciousness that allows a person to escape the perpetual cycle of life, death and rebirth. While this belief is far from extinct in modern society, it is something that a significant proportion of those that take an interest in meditation have no particular interest in. In a world of pressure, stress, interconnected social networks both tangible and virtual and complex social and political issues, meditation has grown in popularity for some of the benefits it yields on the way to achieving that most elusive ultimate state of consciousness.

Scientific evidence of the positive changes meditation can bring about in the lives of modern citizens has been an intrinsic part of its recent surge in popularity. The holistic practice of meditation is a lifelong commitment, but different approaches to it, breaking the whole into its parts, can have positive effects on people's inner peace, ability to cope with new challenges, mental health issues, overcoming of personal obstacles and capacity for love and compassion. In this book, we have taken a step-by-step approach to exploring the many facets of meditation, ways the beginner can access them, and the incredibly spiritual gains one can experience by linking all the pieces together.

There isn't a person alive today who couldn't benefit from meditation, and for some the only obstacles to incorporating it into their lives are closed-mindedness to its relevance in today's society, and misconception that they don't have the time for it. Generation by generation, many of the most prominent global difficulties faced by humankind stem from crises of identity, inability to cope with the pressures and corruption they perceive among their surroundings, and trappings of a psychological complexity that is wired to self-destruct, often without any means of recognizing or tending to the negative thought processes that cause such suffering.

There are few people more attuned to the suffering of living creatures than those who engage in serious meditation. Not only does it promote self-healing and empowerment, it also intrinsically motivates practitioners to act with compassion and empathy towards all living things in the world. Bringing meditation into your life is a big step, and will lead to a complex commitment of you incorporate it into your life in the correct way, but it is a commitment you will be glad you made once its benefits begin to wash over you.